*This Journal belongs to:*

_____

There is a saying – you can't manage what you don't measure.

Measuring your intake helps you manage your output.

A healthier inside makes for a more attractive outside.

Become your own Boss today, by managing what you eat, and how you use those calories

# Tips for using a habit tracker

- **Why**

  - Here a five compelling reasons.
  - 1. It creates a visual cue that can remind you to act.
  - 2. It is motivating to see the progress you are making.
  - 3. It motivates you to continue.
  - 4. It provides immediate satisfaction.
  - 5. Finally, tracking feels rewarding
  - Tracking specific habits also helps keep you focused on the process rather
  - than the result.

- **What**
  -
- **Common habits to track:**
  - meditate
  - write 1 thing I'm grateful for
  - Exercise
  - Walk the dog

- **When**
  - Anytime you remember really but it has been found for some that )
  -

# Habit Tracker

Month _____
Year

| Day | Write in Journal | Meditate | Exercise | | | | | | | | | | | | | |
|---|---|---|---|---|---|---|---|---|---|---|---|---|---|---|---|---|
| 1 | �in | | ▪ | | | | | | | | | | | | | |
| 2 | | ▪ | | | | | | | | | | | | | | |
| 3 | ▪ | ▪ | ▪ | | | | | | | | | | | | | |
| 4 | | ▪ | | | | | | | | | | | | | | |
| 5 | ▪ | | ▪ | | | | | | | | | | | | | |
| 6 | | ▪ | ▪ | | | | | | | | | | | | | |
| 7 | ▪ | | | | | | | | | | | | | | | |
| 8 | | | | | | | | | | | | | | | | |
| 9 | | | | | | | | | | | | | | | | |
| 10 | | | | | | | | | | | | | | | | |
| 11 | | | | | | | | | | | | | | | | |
| 12 | | | | | | | | | | | | | | | | |
| 13 | | | | | | | | | | | | | | | | |
| 14 | | | | | | | | | | | | | | | | |
| 15 | | | | | | | | | | | | | | | | |
| 16 | | | | | | | | | | | | | | | | |
| 17 | | | | | | | | | | | | | | | | |
| 18 | | | | | | | | | | | | | | | | |
| 19 | | | | | | | | | | | | | | | | |
| 20 | | | | | | | | | | | | | | | | |
| 21 | | | | | | | | | | | | | | | | |
| 22 | | | | | | | | | | | | | | | | |
| 23 | | | | | | | | | | | | | | | | |
| 24 | | | | | | | | | | | | | | | | |
| 25 | | | | | | | | | | | | | | | | |
| 26 | | | | | | | | | | | | | | | | |
| 27 | | | | | | | | | | | | | | | | |
| 28 | | | | | | | | | | | | | | | | |
| 29 | | | | | | | | | | | | | | | | |
| 30 | | | | | | | | | | | | | | | | |
| 31 | | | | | | | | | | | | | | | | |

# Habit
# Tracker

y

Notes:

| Date | | S  M  T  W  T  F  S | |
|---|---|---|---|
| **Breakfast** | | Amount | Calories (kcal) |
| | | | |
| | | | |
| | | | |
| | | | |
| | | | |
| | | Total | |
| **Snack** | | Amount | Calories (kcal) |
| | | | |
| | | | |
| | | | |
| | | | |
| | | | |
| | | | |
| | | Total | |
| **Lunch** | | Amount | Calories (kcal) |
| | | | |
| | | | |
| | | | |
| | | | |
| | | | |
| | | Total | |

| Snack | Amount | Calories (kcal) |
|---|---|---|
| | | |
| | | |
| | | |
| | Total | |
| Dinner | Amount | Calories (kcal) |
| | | |
| | | |
| | | |
| | | |
| | | |
| | | |
| | Total | |
| Snack | Amount | Calories (kcal) |
| | | |
| | | |
| | | |
| | Total | |
| Exercise | Duration | Calories burned (kcal) |
| | | |
| | | |
| | | |
| Water | | Fruit & Veggies | |

# Notes:

| Date | S M T W T F S | |
|---|---|---|
| **Breakfast** | Amount | Calories (kcal) |
| | | |
| | | |
| | | |
| | | |
| | | |
| | Total | |
| **Snack** | Amount | Calories (kcal) |
| | | |
| | | |
| | | |
| | | |
| | | |
| | | |
| | Total | |
| **Lunch** | Amount | Calories (kcal) |
| | | |
| | | |
| | | |
| | | |
| | | |
| | | |
| | Total | |

| Snack | Amount | Calories (kcal) |
|---|---|---|
| | | |
| | | |
| | | |
| | Total | |
| Dinner | Amount | Calories (kcal) |
| | | |
| | | |
| | | |
| | | |
| | | |
| | | |
| | | |
| | Total | |
| Snack | Amount | Calories (kcal) |
| | | |
| | | |
| | | |
| | Total | |
| Exercise | Duration | Calories burned (kcal) |
| | | |
| | | |
| | | |

| Water | | | | | | | | Fruit & Veggies | | | | | | | |
|---|---|---|---|---|---|---|---|---|---|---|---|---|---|---|---|

Notes:

| Date | | S  M  T  W  T  F  S | |
|---|---|---|---|
| **Breakfast** | | Amount | Calories (kcal) |
| | | | |
| | | | |
| | | | |
| | | | |
| | | | |
| | | Total | |
| **Snack** | | Amount | Calories (kcal) |
| | | | |
| | | | |
| | | | |
| | | | |
| | | | |
| | | | |
| | | Total | |
| **Lunch** | | Amount | Calories (kcal) |
| | | | |
| | | | |
| | | | |
| | | | |
| | | | |
| | | Total | |

| Snack | Amount | Calories (kcal) |
|---|---|---|
|  |  |  |
|  |  |  |
|  |  |  |
|  | Total |  |
| **Dinner** | Amount | Calories (kcal) |
|  |  |  |
|  |  |  |
|  |  |  |
|  |  |  |
|  |  |  |
|  |  |  |
|  |  |  |
|  | Total |  |
| **Snack** | Amount | Calories (kcal) |
|  |  |  |
|  |  |  |
|  |  |  |
|  | Total |  |
| **Exercise** | Duration | Calories burned (kcal) |
|  |  |  |
|  |  |  |
|  |  |  |
| **Water** | Fruit & Veggies |  |

Notes:

| Date | | S M T W T F S | |
|---|---|---|---|
| **Breakfast** | | Amount | Calories (kcal) |
| | | | |
| | | | |
| | | | |
| | | | |
| | | | |
| | | Total | |
| **Snack** | | Amount | Calories (kcal) |
| | | | |
| | | | |
| | | | |
| | | | |
| | | | |
| | | | |
| | | Total | |
| **Lunch** | | Amount | Calories (kcal) |
| | | | |
| | | | |
| | | | |
| | | | |
| | | | |
| | | | |
| | | Total | |

| Snack | Amount | Calories (kcal) |
|---|---|---|
| | | |
| | | |
| | | |
| | Total | |
| **Dinner** | Amount | Calories (kcal) |
| | | |
| | | |
| | | |
| | | |
| | | |
| | | |
| | Total | |
| **Snack** | Amount | Calories (kcal) |
| | | |
| | | |
| | | |
| | Total | |
| **Exercise** | Duration | Calories burned (kcal) |
| | | |
| | | |
| | | |

| Water | | | | | | | | Fruit & Veggies | | | | | | | | |
|---|---|---|---|---|---|---|---|---|---|---|---|---|---|---|---|---|

Notes:

| Date | S M T W T F S | |
|---|---|---|
| **Breakfast** | Amount | Calories (kcal) |
| | | |
| | | |
| | | |
| | | |
| | | |
| | Total | |
| **Snack** | Amount | Calories (kcal) |
| | | |
| | | |
| | | |
| | | |
| | | |
| | | |
| | Total | |
| **Lunch** | Amount | Calories (kcal) |
| | | |
| | | |
| | | |
| | | |
| | | |
| | | |
| | Total | |

| Snack | Amount | Calories (kcal) |
|---|---|---|
| | | |
| | | |
| | | |
| | Total | |
| Dinner | Amount | Calories (kcal) |
| | | |
| | | |
| | | |
| | | |
| | | |
| | | |
| | | |
| | Total | |
| Snack | Amount | Calories (kcal) |
| | | |
| | | |
| | | |
| | Total | |
| Exercise | Duration | Calories burned (kcal) |
| | | |
| | | |
| | | |
| Water | | Fruit & Veggies | |

Notes:

| Date | | S M T W T F S | |
|---|---|---|---|
| **Breakfast** | Amount | | Calories (kcal) |
| | | | |
| | | | |
| | | | |
| | | | |
| | | | |
| | Total | | |
| **Snack** | Amount | | Calories (kcal) |
| | | | |
| | | | |
| | | | |
| | | | |
| | | | |
| | | | |
| | Total | | |
| **Lunch** | Amount | | Calories (kcal) |
| | | | |
| | | | |
| | | | |
| | | | |
| | | | |
| | | | |
| | Total | | |

| Snack | Amount | Calories (kcal) |
|---|---|---|
|  |  |  |
|  |  |  |
|  |  |  |
|  | Total |  |

| Dinner | Amount | Calories (kcal) |
|---|---|---|
|  |  |  |
|  |  |  |
|  |  |  |
|  |  |  |
|  |  |  |
|  |  |  |
|  | Total |  |

| Snack | Amount | Calories (kcal) |
|---|---|---|
|  |  |  |
|  |  |  |
|  |  |  |
|  | Total |  |

| Exercise | Duration | Calories burned (kcal) |
|---|---|---|
|  |  |  |
|  |  |  |
|  |  |  |

| Water |  |  |  |  |  |  |  |  | Fruit & Veggies |  |  |  |  |  |  |  |  |
|---|---|---|---|---|---|---|---|---|---|---|---|---|---|---|---|---|---|

Notes:

| Date | S M T W T F S | |
|---|---|---|
| **Breakfast** | Amount | Calories (kcal) |
| | | |
| | | |
| | | |
| | | |
| | | |
| | Total | |
| **Snack** | Amount | Calories (kcal) |
| | | |
| | | |
| | | |
| | | |
| | | |
| | | |
| | Total | |
| **Lunch** | Amount | Calories (kcal) |
| | | |
| | | |
| | | |
| | | |
| | | |
| | | |
| | Total | |

| Snack | Amount | Calories (kcal) |
|---|---|---|
| | | |
| | | |
| | | |
| | Total | |
| Dinner | Amount | Calories (kcal) |
| | | |
| | | |
| | | |
| | | |
| | | |
| | | |
| | | |
| | Total | |
| Snack | Amount | Calories (kcal) |
| | | |
| | | |
| | | |
| | Total | |
| Exercise | Duration | Calories burned (kcal) |
| | | |
| | | |
| | | |

| Water | | | | | | | | Fruit & Veggies | | | | | | | |
|---|---|---|---|---|---|---|---|---|---|---|---|---|---|---|---|

Notes:

| Date | | S  M  T  W  T  F  S | |
|---|---|---|---|
| **Breakfast** | Amount | | Calories (kcal) |
| | | | |
| | | | |
| | | | |
| | | | |
| | Total | | |
| **Snack** | Amount | | Calories (kcal) |
| | | | |
| | | | |
| | | | |
| | | | |
| | | | |
| | | | |
| | Total | | |
| **Lunch** | Amount | | Calories (kcal) |
| | | | |
| | | | |
| | | | |
| | | | |
| | | | |
| | | | |
| | Total | | |

| Snack | Amount | Calories (kcal) |
|---|---|---|
|  |  |  |
|  |  |  |
|  | Total |  |

| Dinner | Amount | Calories (kcal) |
|---|---|---|
|  |  |  |
|  |  |  |
|  |  |  |
|  |  |  |
|  |  |  |
|  | Total |  |

| Snack | Amount | Calories (kcal) |
|---|---|---|
|  |  |  |
|  |  |  |
|  | Total |  |

| Exercise | Duration | Calories burned (kcal) |
|---|---|---|
|  |  |  |
|  |  |  |
|  |  |  |

| Water |  |  |  |  |  |  |  | Fruit & Veggies |  |  |  |  |  |  |  |
|---|---|---|---|---|---|---|---|---|---|---|---|---|---|---|---|

Notes:

| Date | S M T W T F S | |
|---|---|---|
| **Breakfast** | Amount | Calories (kcal) |
| | | |
| | | |
| | | |
| | | |
| | | |
| | Total | |
| **Snack** | Amount | Calories (kcal) |
| | | |
| | | |
| | | |
| | | |
| | | |
| | Total | |
| **Lunch** | Amount | Calories (kcal) |
| | | |
| | | |
| | | |
| | | |
| | | |
| | Total | |

| Snack | Amount | Calories (kcal) |
|---|---|---|
| | | |
| | | |
| | | |
| | Total | |
| **Dinner** | Amount | Calories (kcal) |
| | | |
| | | |
| | | |
| | | |
| | | |
| | | |
| | | |
| | Total | |
| **Snack** | Amount | Calories (kcal) |
| | | |
| | | |
| | | |
| | Total | |
| **Exercise** | Duration | Calories burned (kcal) |
| | | |
| | | |
| | | |
| **Water** | | | | | | | | | **Fruit & Veggies** | | | | | | | | |

# Notes:

| Date | | S  M  T  W  T  F  S | |
|---|---|---|---|
| **Breakfast** | Amount | Calories (kcal) | |
| | | | |
| | | | |
| | | | |
| | | | |
| | Total | | |
| **Snack** | Amount | Calories (kcal) | |
| | | | |
| | | | |
| | | | |
| | | | |
| | | | |
| | | | |
| | Total | | |
| **Lunch** | Amount | Calories (kcal) | |
| | | | |
| | | | |
| | | | |
| | | | |
| | | | |
| | Total | | |

| Snack | Amount | Calories (kcal) |
|---|---|---|
| | | |
| | | |
| | | |
| | Total | |
| **Dinner** | Amount | Calories (kcal) |
| | | |
| | | |
| | | |
| | | |
| | | |
| | | |
| | Total | |
| **Snack** | Amount | Calories (kcal) |
| | | |
| | | |
| | Total | |
| **Exercise** | Duration | Calories burned (kcal) |
| | | |
| | | |
| | | |

| Water | | | | | | | | Fruit & Veggies | | | | | | | |
|---|---|---|---|---|---|---|---|---|---|---|---|---|---|---|---|

Notes:

| Date | S M T W T F S | |
|---|---|---|
| **Breakfast** | Amount | Calories (kcal) |
| | | |
| | | |
| | | |
| | | |
| | | |
| | Total | |
| **Snack** | Amount | Calories (kcal) |
| | | |
| | | |
| | | |
| | | |
| | | |
| | | |
| | Total | |
| **Lunch** | Amount | Calories (kcal) |
| | | |
| | | |
| | | |
| | | |
| | | |
| | | |
| | Total | |

| Snack | Amount | Calories (kcal) |
|---|---|---|
| | | |
| | | |
| | | |
| | Total | |
| **Dinner** | Amount | Calories (kcal) |
| | | |
| | | |
| | | |
| | | |
| | | |
| | | |
| | | |
| | Total | |
| **Snack** | Amount | Calories (kcal) |
| | | |
| | | |
| | | |
| | Total | |
| **Exercise** | Duration | Calories burned (kcal) |
| | | |
| | | |
| | | |

| Water | | | | | | | | | | Fruit & Veggies | | | | | | | | |
|---|---|---|---|---|---|---|---|---|---|---|---|---|---|---|---|---|---|---|

Notes:

| Date | | S M T W T F S | |
|---|---|---|---|
| **Breakfast** | Amount | | Calories (kcal) |
| | | | |
| | | | |
| | | | |
| | | | |
| | Total | | |
| **Snack** | Amount | | Calories (kcal) |
| | | | |
| | | | |
| | | | |
| | | | |
| | | | |
| | Total | | |
| **Lunch** | Amount | | Calories (kcal) |
| | | | |
| | | | |
| | | | |
| | | | |
| | | | |
| | | | |
| | Total | | |

| Snack | Amount | Calories (kcal) |
|---|---|---|
|  |  |  |
|  |  |  |
|  |  |  |
|  | Total |  |

| Dinner | Amount | Calories (kcal) |
|---|---|---|
|  |  |  |
|  |  |  |
|  |  |  |
|  |  |  |
|  |  |  |
|  |  |  |
|  | Total |  |

| Snack | Amount | Calories (kcal) |
|---|---|---|
|  |  |  |
|  |  |  |
|  | Total |  |

| Exercise | Duration | Calories burned (kcal) |
|---|---|---|
|  |  |  |
|  |  |  |
|  |  |  |

| Water | | | | | | | | Fruit & Veggies | | | | | | | |
|---|---|---|---|---|---|---|---|---|---|---|---|---|---|---|---|

Notes:

| Date | | S M T W T F S | |
|---|---|---|---|
| **Breakfast** | | Amount | Calories (kcal) |
| | | | |
| | | | |
| | | | |
| | | | |
| | | | |
| | | Total | |
| **Snack** | | Amount | Calories (kcal) |
| | | | |
| | | | |
| | | | |
| | | | |
| | | | |
| | | Total | |
| **Lunch** | | Amount | Calories (kcal) |
| | | | |
| | | | |
| | | | |
| | | | |
| | | | |
| | | Total | |

| Snack | Amount | Calories (kcal) |
|---|---|---|
| | | |
| | | |
| | | |
| | Total | |
| **Dinner** | Amount | Calories (kcal) |
| | | |
| | | |
| | | |
| | | |
| | | |
| | | |
| | | |
| | Total | |
| **Snack** | Amount | Calories (kcal) |
| | | |
| | | |
| | | |
| | Total | |
| **Exercise** | Duration | Calories burned (kcal) |
| | | |
| | | |
| | | |
| **Water** | Fruit & Veggies | |

Notes:

| Date | | S M T W T F S | |
|---|---|---|---|
| **Breakfast** | | Amount | Calories (kcal) |
| | | | |
| | | | |
| | | | |
| | | | |
| | | Total | |
| **Snack** | | Amount | Calories (kcal) |
| | | | |
| | | | |
| | | | |
| | | | |
| | | | |
| | | | |
| | | Total | |
| **Lunch** | | Amount | Calories (kcal) |
| | | | |
| | | | |
| | | | |
| | | | |
| | | | |
| | | | |
| | | Total | |

| Snack | Amount | Calories (kcal) |
|---|---|---|
| | | |
| | | |
| | | |
| | Total | |
| **Dinner** | Amount | Calories (kcal) |
| | | |
| | | |
| | | |
| | | |
| | | |
| | | |
| | Total | |
| **Snack** | Amount | Calories (kcal) |
| | | |
| | | |
| | Total | |
| **Exercise** | Duration | Calories burned (kcal) |
| | | |
| | | |
| | | |

| Water | | | | | | | | Fruit & Veggies | | | | | | | |
|---|---|---|---|---|---|---|---|---|---|---|---|---|---|---|---|

Notes:

| Date | | S  M  T  W  T  F  S | |
|---|---|---|---|
| **Breakfast** | | Amount | Calories (kcal) |
| | | | |
| | | | |
| | | | |
| | | | |
| | | | |
| | | Total | |
| **Snack** | | Amount | Calories (kcal) |
| | | | |
| | | | |
| | | | |
| | | | |
| | | | |
| | | Total | |
| **Lunch** | | Amount | Calories (kcal) |
| | | | |
| | | | |
| | | | |
| | | | |
| | | | |
| | | Total | |

| Snack | Amount | Calories (kcal) |
|---|---|---|
| | | |
| | | |
| | | |
| | Total | |
| Dinner | Amount | Calories (kcal) |
| | | |
| | | |
| | | |
| | | |
| | | |
| | | |
| | | |
| | Total | |
| Snack | Amount | Calories (kcal) |
| | | |
| | | |
| | Total | |
| Exercise | Duration | Calories burned (kcal) |
| | | |
| | | |
| | | |
| Water | | Fruit & Veggies | |

Notes:

| Date | | S  M  T  W  T  F  S |
|---|---|---|
| **Breakfast** | Amount | Calories (kcal) |
| | | |
| | | |
| | | |
| | | |
| | | |
| | Total | |
| **Snack** | Amount | Calories (kcal) |
| | | |
| | | |
| | | |
| | | |
| | | |
| | | |
| | Total | |
| **Lunch** | Amount | Calories (kcal) |
| | | |
| | | |
| | | |
| | | |
| | | |
| | | |
| | Total | |

| Snack | Amount | Calories (kcal) |
|---|---|---|
|  |  |  |
|  |  |  |
|  |  |  |
|  | Total |  |
| **Dinner** | Amount | Calories (kcal) |
|  |  |  |
|  |  |  |
|  |  |  |
|  |  |  |
|  |  |  |
|  |  |  |
|  | Total |  |
| **Snack** | Amount | Calories (kcal) |
|  |  |  |
|  |  |  |
|  | Total |  |
| **Exercise** | Duration | Calories burned (kcal) |
|  |  |  |
|  |  |  |
|  |  |  |

| Water | | | | | | | | Fruit & Veggies | | | | | | | |
|---|---|---|---|---|---|---|---|---|---|---|---|---|---|---|---|

Notes:

| Date | S M T W T F S | |
|---|---|---|
| **Breakfast** | Amount | Calories (kcal) |
| | | |
| | | |
| | | |
| | | |
| | Total | |
| **Snack** | Amount | Calories (kcal) |
| | | |
| | | |
| | | |
| | | |
| | | |
| | Total | |
| **Lunch** | Amount | Calories (kcal) |
| | | |
| | | |
| | | |
| | | |
| | | |
| | Total | |

| Snack | Amount | Calories (kcal) |
|---|---|---|
|  |  |  |
|  |  |  |
|  |  |  |
|  | Total |  |
| Dinner | Amount | Calories (kcal) |
|  |  |  |
|  |  |  |
|  |  |  |
|  |  |  |
|  |  |  |
|  |  |  |
|  |  |  |
|  | Total |  |
| Snack | Amount | Calories (kcal) |
|  |  |  |
|  |  |  |
|  |  |  |
|  | Total |  |
| Exercise | Duration | Calories burned (kcal) |
|  |  |  |
|  |  |  |
|  |  |  |
| Water | | | | | | | | Fruit & Veggies | | | | | | | |

Notes:

| Date | | S   M   T   W   T   F   S | |
|---|---|---|---|
| **Breakfast** | Amount | Calories (kcal) | |
| | | | |
| | | | |
| | | | |
| | | | |
| | | | |
| | Total | | |
| **Snack** | Amount | Calories (kcal) | |
| | | | |
| | | | |
| | | | |
| | | | |
| | | | |
| | | | |
| | Total | | |
| **Lunch** | Amount | Calories (kcal) | |
| | | | |
| | | | |
| | | | |
| | | | |
| | | | |
| | | | |
| | Total | | |

| Snack | Amount | Calories (kcal) |
|---|---|---|
| | | |
| | | |
| | | |
| | Total | |
| **Dinner** | Amount | Calories (kcal) |
| | | |
| | | |
| | | |
| | | |
| | | |
| | | |
| | Total | |
| **Snack** | Amount | Calories (kcal) |
| | | |
| | | |
| | Total | |
| **Exercise** | Duration | Calories burned (kcal) |
| | | |
| | | |
| | | |
| **Water** | Fruit & Veggies | |

## Notes:

| Date | S M T W T F S | |
|---|---|---|
| **Breakfast** | Amount | Calories (kcal) |
| | | |
| | | |
| | | |
| | | |
| | Total | |
| **Snack** | Amount | Calories (kcal) |
| | | |
| | | |
| | | |
| | | |
| | | |
| | Total | |
| **Lunch** | Amount | Calories (kcal) |
| | | |
| | | |
| | | |
| | | |
| | | |
| | Total | |

| Snack | Amount | Calories (kcal) |
|---|---|---|
| | | |
| | | |
| | | |
| | Total | |
| Dinner | Amount | Calories (kcal) |
| | | |
| | | |
| | | |
| | | |
| | | |
| | | |
| | Total | |
| Snack | Amount | Calories (kcal) |
| | | |
| | | |
| | | |
| | Total | |
| Exercise | Duration | Calories burned (kcal) |
| | | |
| | | |
| | | |
| Water | | Fruit & Veggies | |

Notes:

| Date | S M T W T F S | |
|---|---|---|
| **Breakfast** | Amount | Calories (kcal) |
| | | |
| | | |
| | | |
| | | |
| | | |
| | Total | |
| **Snack** | Amount | Calories (kcal) |
| | | |
| | | |
| | | |
| | | |
| | | |
| | | |
| | Total | |
| **Lunch** | Amount | Calories (kcal) |
| | | |
| | | |
| | | |
| | | |
| | | |
| | | |
| | Total | |

| Snack | Amount | Calories (kcal) |
|---|---|---|
| | | |
| | | |
| | | |
| | Total | |
| **Dinner** | Amount | Calories (kcal) |
| | | |
| | | |
| | | |
| | | |
| | | |
| | | |
| | Total | |
| **Snack** | Amount | Calories (kcal) |
| | | |
| | | |
| | | |
| | Total | |
| **Exercise** | Duration | Calories burned (kcal) |
| | | |
| | | |
| | | |
| **Water** | Fruit & Veggies | |

Notes:

| Date | | S M T W T F S | |
|---|---|---|---|
| **Breakfast** | | Amount | Calories (kcal) |
| | | | |
| | | | |
| | | | |
| | | | |
| | | | |
| | | Total | |
| **Snack** | | Amount | Calories (kcal) |
| | | | |
| | | | |
| | | | |
| | | | |
| | | | |
| | | | |
| | | Total | |
| **Lunch** | | Amount | Calories (kcal) |
| | | | |
| | | | |
| | | | |
| | | | |
| | | | |
| | | | |
| | | Total | |

| Snack | Amount | Calories (kcal) |
|---|---|---|
|  |  |  |
|  |  |  |
|  |  |  |
|  | Total |  |
| **Dinner** | Amount | Calories (kcal) |
|  |  |  |
|  |  |  |
|  |  |  |
|  |  |  |
|  |  |  |
|  |  |  |
|  | Total |  |
| **Snack** | Amount | Calories (kcal) |
|  |  |  |
|  |  |  |
|  |  |  |
|  | Total |  |
| **Exercise** | Duration | Calories burned (kcal) |
|  |  |  |
|  |  |  |
|  |  |  |
| **Water** | Fruit & Veggies |  |

Notes:

| Date | | S M T W T F S | |
|---|---|---|---|
| **Breakfast** | Amount | | Calories (kcal) |
| | | | |
| | | | |
| | | | |
| | | | |
| | | | |
| | Total | | |
| **Snack** | Amount | | Calories (kcal) |
| | | | |
| | | | |
| | | | |
| | | | |
| | | | |
| | | | |
| | Total | | |
| **Lunch** | Amount | | Calories (kcal) |
| | | | |
| | | | |
| | | | |
| | | | |
| | | | |
| | | | |
| | Total | | |

| Snack | Amount | Calories (kcal) |
|---|---|---|
| | | |
| | | |
| | Total | |
| Dinner | Amount | Calories (kcal) |
| | | |
| | | |
| | | |
| | | |
| | | |
| | | |
| | Total | |
| Snack | Amount | Calories (kcal) |
| | | |
| | | |
| | | |
| | Total | |
| Exercise | Duration | Calories burned (kcal) |
| | | |
| | | |
| | | |

| Water | | | | | | | | | Fruit & Veggies | | | | | | | |
|---|---|---|---|---|---|---|---|---|---|---|---|---|---|---|---|---|
| | | | | | | | | | | | | | | | | |

Notes:

| Date | | S  M  T  W  T  F  S | |
|---|---|---|---|
| **Breakfast** | | Amount | Calories (kcal) |
| | | | |
| | | | |
| | | | |
| | | | |
| | | | |
| | | Total | |
| **Snack** | | Amount | Calories (kcal) |
| | | | |
| | | | |
| | | | |
| | | | |
| | | | |
| | | Total | |
| **Lunch** | | Amount | Calories (kcal) |
| | | | |
| | | | |
| | | | |
| | | | |
| | | | |
| | | Total | |

| Snack | Amount | Calories (kcal) |
|---|---|---|
| | | |
| | | |
| | | |
| | Total | |
| **Dinner** | Amount | Calories (kcal) |
| | | |
| | | |
| | | |
| | | |
| | | |
| | | |
| | | |
| | Total | |
| **Snack** | Amount | Calories (kcal) |
| | | |
| | | |
| | | |
| | Total | |
| **Exercise** | Duration | Calories burned (kcal) |
| | | |
| | | |
| | | |
| **Water** | | | | | | | | | Fruit & Veggies | | | | | | | | |

# Notes:

| Date | | S M T W T F S | |
|---|---|---|---|
| **Breakfast** | | Amount | Calories (kcal) |
| | | | |
| | | | |
| | | | |
| | | | |
| | | | |
| | | Total | |
| **Snack** | | Amount | Calories (kcal) |
| | | | |
| | | | |
| | | | |
| | | | |
| | | | |
| | | | |
| | | Total | |
| **Lunch** | | Amount | Calories (kcal) |
| | | | |
| | | | |
| | | | |
| | | | |
| | | | |
| | | | |
| | | Total | |

| Snack | Amount | Calories (kcal) |
|---|---|---|
| | | |
| | | |
| | | |
| | Total | |
| **Dinner** | Amount | Calories (kcal) |
| | | |
| | | |
| | | |
| | | |
| | | |
| | | |
| | | |
| | Total | |
| **Snack** | Amount | Calories (kcal) |
| | | |
| | | |
| | | |
| | Total | |
| **Exercise** | Duration | Calories burned (kcal) |
| | | |
| | | |
| | | |

| Water | | | | | | | Fruit & Veggies | | | | | | | |
|---|---|---|---|---|---|---|---|---|---|---|---|---|---|---|

Notes:

| Date | | S  M  T  W  T  F  S | |
|---|---|---|---|
| **Breakfast** | | Amount | Calories (kcal) |
| | | | |
| | | | |
| | | | |
| | | | |
| | | Total | |
| **Snack** | | Amount | Calories (kcal) |
| | | | |
| | | | |
| | | | |
| | | | |
| | | | |
| | | Total | |
| **Lunch** | | Amount | Calories (kcal) |
| | | | |
| | | | |
| | | | |
| | | | |
| | | | |
| | | Total | |

| Snack | Amount | Calories (kcal) |
|---|---|---|
| | | |
| | | |
| | | |
| | Total | |
| Dinner | Amount | Calories (kcal) |
| | | |
| | | |
| | | |
| | | |
| | | |
| | | |
| | | |
| | Total | |
| Snack | Amount | Calories (kcal) |
| | | |
| | | |
| | | |
| | Total | |
| Exercise | Duration | Calories burned (kcal) |
| | | |
| | | |
| | | |

| Water | | | | | | | | | Fruit & Veggies | | | | | | | | |
|---|---|---|---|---|---|---|---|---|---|---|---|---|---|---|---|---|---|

Notes:

| Date | S  M  T  W  T  F  S | |
|---|---|---|
| **Breakfast** | Amount | Calories (kcal) |
| | | |
| | | |
| | | |
| | | |
| | | |
| | Total | |
| **Snack** | Amount | Calories (kcal) |
| | | |
| | | |
| | | |
| | | |
| | | |
| | | |
| | Total | |
| **Lunch** | Amount | Calories (kcal) |
| | | |
| | | |
| | | |
| | | |
| | | |
| | | |
| | Total | |

| Snack | Amount | Calories (kcal) |
|---|---|---|
|  |  |  |
|  |  |  |
|  |  |  |
|  | Total |  |
| **Dinner** | Amount | Calories (kcal) |
|  |  |  |
|  |  |  |
|  |  |  |
|  |  |  |
|  |  |  |
|  |  |  |
|  | Total |  |
| **Snack** | Amount | Calories (kcal) |
|  |  |  |
|  |  |  |
|  |  |  |
|  | Total |  |
| **Exercise** | Duration | Calories burned (kcal) |
|  |  |  |
|  |  |  |
|  |  |  |
| **Water** | Fruit & Veggies |  |

Notes:

| Date | | S M T W T F S | |
|---|---|---|---|
| **Breakfast** | | Amount | Calories (kcal) |
| | | | |
| | | | |
| | | | |
| | | | |
| | | Total | |
| **Snack** | | Amount | Calories (kcal) |
| | | | |
| | | | |
| | | | |
| | | | |
| | | | |
| | | Total | |
| **Lunch** | | Amount | Calories (kcal) |
| | | | |
| | | | |
| | | | |
| | | | |
| | | | |
| | | Total | |

| Snack | Amount | Calories (kcal) |
|---|---|---|
| | | |
| | | |
| | | |
| | Total | |
| **Dinner** | Amount | Calories (kcal) |
| | | |
| | | |
| | | |
| | | |
| | | |
| | | |
| | | |
| | Total | |
| **Snack** | Amount | Calories (kcal) |
| | | |
| | | |
| | | |
| | Total | |
| **Exercise** | Duration | Calories burned (kcal) |
| | | |
| | | |
| | | |
| **Water** | Fruit & Veggies | |

Notes:

| Date | S M T W T F S | |
|---|---|---|
| **Breakfast** | Amount | Calories (kcal) |
| | | |
| | | |
| | | |
| | | |
| | Total | |
| **Snack** | Amount | Calories (kcal) |
| | | |
| | | |
| | | |
| | | |
| | | |
| | | |
| | Total | |
| **Lunch** | Amount | Calories (kcal) |
| | | |
| | | |
| | | |
| | | |
| | | |
| | | |
| | Total | |

| Snack | Amount | Calories (kcal) |
|---|---|---|
| | | |
| | | |
| | | |
| | Total | |
| **Dinner** | Amount | Calories (kcal) |
| | | |
| | | |
| | | |
| | | |
| | | |
| | | |
| | | |
| | Total | |
| **Snack** | Amount | Calories (kcal) |
| | | |
| | | |
| | | |
| | Total | |
| **Exercise** | Duration | Calories burned (kcal) |
| | | |
| | | |
| | | |

| Water | | | | | | | | Fruit & Veggies | | | | | | | |
|---|---|---|---|---|---|---|---|---|---|---|---|---|---|---|---|

Notes:

| Date | | S  M  T  W  T  F  S | |
|---|---|---|---|
| **Breakfast** | | Amount | Calories (kcal) |
| | | | |
| | | | |
| | | | |
| | | | |
| | | | |
| | | Total | |
| **Snack** | | Amount | Calories (kcal) |
| | | | |
| | | | |
| | | | |
| | | | |
| | | | |
| | | | |
| | | Total | |
| **Lunch** | | Amount | Calories (kcal) |
| | | | |
| | | | |
| | | | |
| | | | |
| | | | |
| | | | |
| | | Total | |

| Snack | Amount | Calories (kcal) |
|---|---|---|
|  |  |  |
|  |  |  |
|  |  |  |
|  | Total |  |
| Dinner | Amount | Calories (kcal) |
|  |  |  |
|  |  |  |
|  |  |  |
|  |  |  |
|  |  |  |
|  |  |  |
|  |  |  |
|  | Total |  |
| Snack | Amount | Calories (kcal) |
|  |  |  |
|  |  |  |
|  |  |  |
|  | Total |  |
| Exercise | Duration | Calories burned (kcal) |
|  |  |  |
|  |  |  |
|  |  |  |
| Water |  | Fruit & Veggies |

## Notes:

| Date | S M T W T F S | |
|---|---|---|
| **Breakfast** | Amount | Calories (kcal) |
| | | |
| | | |
| | | |
| | | |
| | | |
| | Total | |
| **Snack** | Amount | Calories (kcal) |
| | | |
| | | |
| | | |
| | | |
| | | |
| | | |
| | Total | |
| **Lunch** | Amount | Calories (kcal) |
| | | |
| | | |
| | | |
| | | |
| | | |
| | Total | |

| Snack | Amount | Calories (kcal) |
|---|---|---|
| | | |
| | | |
| | | |
| | Total | |
| **Dinner** | Amount | Calories (kcal) |
| | | |
| | | |
| | | |
| | | |
| | | |
| | | |
| | | |
| | Total | |
| **Snack** | Amount | Calories (kcal) |
| | | |
| | | |
| | | |
| | Total | |
| **Exercise** | Duration | Calories burned (kcal) |
| | | |
| | | |
| | | |
| **Water** | | | | | | | | **Fruit & Veggies** | | | | | | | | |

Notes:

| Date | S M T W T F S | |
|---|---|---|
| **Breakfast** | Amount | Calories (kcal) |
| | | |
| | | |
| | | |
| | | |
| | | |
| | Total | |
| **Snack** | Amount | Calories (kcal) |
| | | |
| | | |
| | | |
| | | |
| | | |
| | | |
| | Total | |
| **Lunch** | Amount | Calories (kcal) |
| | | |
| | | |
| | | |
| | | |
| | | |
| | | |
| | Total | |

| Snack | Amount | Calories (kcal) |
|---|---|---|
| | | |
| | | |
| | | |
| | Total | |
| Dinner | Amount | Calories (kcal) |
| | | |
| | | |
| | | |
| | | |
| | | |
| | | |
| | | |
| | Total | |
| Snack | Amount | Calories (kcal) |
| | | |
| | | |
| | | |
| | Total | |
| Exercise | Duration | Calories burned (kcal) |
| | | |
| | | |
| | | |

| Water | | | | | | | | | Fruit & Veggies | | | | | | | |
|---|---|---|---|---|---|---|---|---|---|---|---|---|---|---|---|---|

Notes:

| Date | | S  M  T  W  T  F  S | |
|---|---|---|---|
| **Breakfast** | | Amount | Calories (kcal) |
| | | | |
| | | | |
| | | | |
| | | | |
| | | | |
| | | Total | |
| **Snack** | | Amount | Calories (kcal) |
| | | | |
| | | | |
| | | | |
| | | | |
| | | | |
| | | | |
| | | Total | |
| **Lunch** | | Amount | Calories (kcal) |
| | | | |
| | | | |
| | | | |
| | | | |
| | | | |
| | | | |
| | | Total | |

| Snack | Amount | Calories (kcal) |
|---|---|---|
| | | |
| | | |
| | | |
| | Total | |
| **Dinner** | Amount | Calories (kcal) |
| | | |
| | | |
| | | |
| | | |
| | | |
| | | |
| | | |
| | Total | |
| **Snack** | Amount | Calories (kcal) |
| | | |
| | | |
| | | |
| | Total | |
| **Exercise** | Duration | Calories burned (kcal) |
| | | |
| | | |
| | | |
| **Water** | | | | | | | | Fruit & Veggies | | | | | | | | |

# Notes:

| Date | S M T W T F S | |
|---|---|---|
| **Breakfast** | Amount | Calories (kcal) |
| | | |
| | | |
| | | |
| | | |
| | | |
| | Total | |
| **Snack** | Amount | Calories (kcal) |
| | | |
| | | |
| | | |
| | | |
| | | |
| | | |
| | Total | |
| **Lunch** | Amount | Calories (kcal) |
| | | |
| | | |
| | | |
| | | |
| | | |
| | | |
| | Total | |

| Snack | Amount | Calories (kcal) |
|---|---|---|
| | | |
| | | |
| | | |
| | Total | |
| **Dinner** | Amount | Calories (kcal) |
| | | |
| | | |
| | | |
| | | |
| | | |
| | | |
| | | |
| | Total | |
| **Snack** | Amount | Calories (kcal) |
| | | |
| | | |
| | | |
| | Total | |
| **Exercise** | Duration | Calories burned (kcal) |
| | | |
| | | |
| | | |
| **Water** | Fruit & Veggies | |

Notes:

| Date | | S M T W T F S | |
|---|---|---|---|
| **Breakfast** | | Amount | Calories (kcal) |
| | | | |
| | | | |
| | | | |
| | | | |
| | | | |
| | | Total | |
| **Snack** | | Amount | Calories (kcal) |
| | | | |
| | | | |
| | | | |
| | | | |
| | | | |
| | | | |
| | | Total | |
| **Lunch** | | Amount | Calories (kcal) |
| | | | |
| | | | |
| | | | |
| | | | |
| | | | |
| | | | |
| | | Total | |

| Snack | Amount | Calories (kcal) |
|---|---|---|
| | | |
| | | |
| | | |
| | Total | |
| **Dinner** | Amount | Calories (kcal) |
| | | |
| | | |
| | | |
| | | |
| | | |
| | | |
| | | |
| | Total | |
| **Snack** | Amount | Calories (kcal) |
| | | |
| | | |
| | | |
| | Total | |
| **Exercise** | Duration | Calories burned (kcal) |
| | | |
| | | |
| | | |
| **Water** | Fruit & Veggies | |

Notes:

| Date | | S M T W T F S | |
|---|---|---|---|
| **Breakfast** | | Amount | Calories (kcal) |
| | | | |
| | | | |
| | | | |
| | | | |
| | | | |
| | | Total | |
| **Snack** | | Amount | Calories (kcal) |
| | | | |
| | | | |
| | | | |
| | | | |
| | | | |
| | | | |
| | | Total | |
| **Lunch** | | Amount | Calories (kcal) |
| | | | |
| | | | |
| | | | |
| | | | |
| | | | |
| | | Total | |

| Snack | Amount | Calories (kcal) |
|---|---|---|
| | | |
| | | |
| | | |
| | Total | |
| **Dinner** | Amount | Calories (kcal) |
| | | |
| | | |
| | | |
| | | |
| | | |
| | | |
| | | |
| | Total | |
| **Snack** | Amount | Calories (kcal) |
| | | |
| | | |
| | | |
| | Total | |
| **Exercise** | Duration | Calories burned (kcal) |
| | | |
| | | |
| | | |
| **Water** | Fruit & Veggies | |

Notes:

| Date | | S  M  T  W  T  F  S | |
|---|---|---|---|
| **Breakfast** | | Amount | Calories (kcal) |
| | | | |
| | | | |
| | | | |
| | | | |
| | | Total | |
| **Snack** | | Amount | Calories (kcal) |
| | | | |
| | | | |
| | | | |
| | | | |
| | | | |
| | | | |
| | | Total | |
| **Lunch** | | Amount | Calories (kcal) |
| | | | |
| | | | |
| | | | |
| | | | |
| | | | |
| | | Total | |

| Snack | Amount | Calories (kcal) |
|---|---|---|
| | | |
| | | |
| | | |
| | Total | |
| **Dinner** | Amount | Calories (kcal) |
| | | |
| | | |
| | | |
| | | |
| | | |
| | | |
| | | |
| | Total | |
| **Snack** | Amount | Calories (kcal) |
| | | |
| | | |
| | | |
| | Total | |
| **Exercise** | Duration | Calories burned (kcal) |
| | | |
| | | |
| | | |
| **Water** | | | | | | | | | **Fruit & Veggies** | | | | | | | | |

## Notes:

| Date | | S  M  T  W  T  F  S | |
|---|---|---|---|
| **Breakfast** | | Amount | Calories (kcal) |
| | | | |
| | | | |
| | | | |
| | | | |
| | | | |
| | | Total | |
| **Snack** | | Amount | Calories (kcal) |
| | | | |
| | | | |
| | | | |
| | | | |
| | | | |
| | | | |
| | | Total | |
| **Lunch** | | Amount | Calories (kcal) |
| | | | |
| | | | |
| | | | |
| | | | |
| | | | |
| | | | |
| | | Total | |

| Snack | Amount | Calories (kcal) |
|---|---|---|
|  |  |  |
|  |  |  |
|  |  |  |
|  | Total |  |
| **Dinner** | Amount | Calories (kcal) |
|  |  |  |
|  |  |  |
|  |  |  |
|  |  |  |
|  |  |  |
|  |  |  |
|  | Total |  |
| **Snack** | Amount | Calories (kcal) |
|  |  |  |
|  |  |  |
|  |  |  |
|  | Total |  |
| **Exercise** | Duration | Calories burned (kcal) |
|  |  |  |
|  |  |  |
|  |  |  |
| **Water** |  | Fruit & Veggies |  |

Notes:

| Date | | S  M  T  W  T  F  S |
|---|---|---|
| **Breakfast** | Amount | Calories (kcal) |
| | | |
| | | |
| | | |
| | | |
| | Total | |
| **Snack** | Amount | Calories (kcal) |
| | | |
| | | |
| | | |
| | | |
| | | |
| | Total | |
| **Lunch** | Amount | Calories (kcal) |
| | | |
| | | |
| | | |
| | | |
| | | |
| | Total | |

| Snack | Amount | Calories (kcal) |
|---|---|---|
| | | |
| | | |
| | | |
| | Total | |
| **Dinner** | Amount | Calories (kcal) |
| | | |
| | | |
| | | |
| | | |
| | | |
| | | |
| | | |
| | Total | |
| **Snack** | Amount | Calories (kcal) |
| | | |
| | | |
| | | |
| | Total | |
| **Exercise** | Duration | Calories burned (kcal) |
| | | |
| | | |
| | | |
| **Water** | | | | | | | | | **Fruit & Veggies** | | | | | | | | | |

Notes:

| Date | | S M T W T F S | |
|---|---|---|---|
| **Breakfast** | | Amount | Calories (kcal) |
| | | | |
| | | | |
| | | | |
| | | | |
| | | | |
| | | Total | |
| **Snack** | | Amount | Calories (kcal) |
| | | | |
| | | | |
| | | | |
| | | | |
| | | | |
| | | | |
| | | Total | |
| **Lunch** | | Amount | Calories (kcal) |
| | | | |
| | | | |
| | | | |
| | | | |
| | | | |
| | | | |
| | | Total | |

| Snack | Amount | Calories (kcal) |
|---|---|---|
| | | |
| | | |
| | | |
| | Total | |
| **Dinner** | Amount | Calories (kcal) |
| | | |
| | | |
| | | |
| | | |
| | | |
| | | |
| | | |
| | Total | |
| **Snack** | Amount | Calories (kcal) |
| | | |
| | | |
| | | |
| | Total | |
| **Exercise** | Duration | Calories burned (kcal) |
| | | |
| | | |
| | | |
| **Water** | | | | | | | | | | Fruit & Veggies | | | | | | | | | |

Notes:

| Date | | S M T W T F S |
|---|---|---|
| **Breakfast** | Amount | Calories (kcal) |
| | | |
| | | |
| | | |
| | | |
| | Total | |
| **Snack** | Amount | Calories (kcal) |
| | | |
| | | |
| | | |
| | | |
| | | |
| | | |
| | Total | |
| **Lunch** | Amount | Calories (kcal) |
| | | |
| | | |
| | | |
| | | |
| | | |
| | | |
| | Total | |

| Snack | Amount | Calories (kcal) |
|---|---|---|
| | | |
| | | |
| | | |
| | Total | |
| **Dinner** | Amount | Calories (kcal) |
| | | |
| | | |
| | | |
| | | |
| | | |
| | | |
| | | |
| | Total | |
| **Snack** | Amount | Calories (kcal) |
| | | |
| | | |
| | | |
| | Total | |
| **Exercise** | Duration | Calories burned (kcal) |
| | | |
| | | |
| | | |
| **Water** | | | | | | | | | Fruit & Veggies | | | | | | | | |